ISBN-13: 978-1717533050
ISBN-10: 1717533051

Any references to historical events, real people, or real places are used fictitiously. Names, characters, and places are products of the author's imagination.

Front Cover Image by: The Murray
Book Design by: The Murray

Published and Printed in the United States of America

First printing edition 2018

www.the.weightlosstreatmentprogram@gmail.com

Table of Contents

Introduction

Hi, my name is Tammey Endevor and I know that weight loss is a huge mile stone in the lives of many. Some want to lose weight to look good, some want to lose weight to impress someone or to fit into their favorite dress or suit that seemed to somehow magically shrink over time and some want to do it to improve their health. Whatever the reason for trying to lose weight it is still one that proves very difficult for many. It may prove to be arduous and stressful at times and many persons give up believing that weight loss is an effort in futility but I would like to let you know that it doesn't have to be so hard.

This is my story, my journey through my fitness life as I tried to lose weight using a collection of programs created, designed or edited by me which points you in the right direction towards weight loss in an easy maintainable way. Never being into fitness and never being a Fitness Trainer or Nutritionist, I have come across many people that needed help just like me, who went to professionals that had the task of designing for them something that works and while they may design a flawless program it doesn't mean that the person following it believes it to be easy. Based on my experiences the information here will direct you towards what I believe would be the best path to take for weight loss.

 I will start out by saying that this method may not work for everyone and while the plans I have used worked for me, it does not mean it will work for you since there are many factors to consider. These factors include sleep, availability of the suggested food items, stress, exercise, body type and your own overall consistency. I can assure you that this plan can help an individual in relatively stable health lose 20 to 30 pounds within 3 months in an easy stress free manner.

While all exercise or nutrition programs rely on individuals' ability to stick to them, this program is no different and would take some will power and drive on your part. Before beginning an exercise program always consult a physician first and always make sure that you are willing to dedicate 3 months of your life to the program for optimal results. In this book, before every level is a simple planner to help you track your work as you read and do the program.

My love for myself and my desire to help individuals meet their goals is my main drive for putting together a work such as this. I hope you enjoy the process and I wish you the best of luck.

Record Your Goals

Name:____

Age:____

Gender:____

Starting Weight:_____________________________________

Realistic Goal: ______________________________________

Words of Encouragement: _____________________________

____

____

____

Level 1

Detox

Hi welcome to level 1. Here I will tell you a little about myself and what made me start on my journey and the first steps I took. I, first of all, am a normal person like any other. There is nothing special about me. I work a regular nine to five. Get up every morning unappreciative of the day, since I had to get out of my precious bed. Ever notice how difficult it is to get out of bed when you got to head out to work? I mean, the thought of going to work makes the bed feel even sweeter. I think that is a master plan.

Anyway, I get out of bed, get ready for work, most times grabbing a slice of toast and coffee, and maybe an apple, you know since I am trying to be healthy and all. I make my way out after taking a lack luster shower and head towards public transportation and deal with my adoring public. The day is pretty boring, meet customers, tell them how much they need one of the products in the store that meets their needs, cash them out and repeat. Pretty much this happens for the entire eight hours of work. The two times of the day I look forward to are lunch, since I can step out and get away from the store and closing time, although I always get that pesky customer that walks in 2 minutes before closing time and that is annoying but I put on a smile and head back home.

Lunch isn't so grand, usually something quick, a burger, chicken sandwich and if I am feeling frisky, a full on meal. Don't you hate when you feel sleepy after a big meal? I mean who does that? Usually a bottle of cool water puts me back in my zone, as dead as that is. Head back to the store to pretend like I want to be there till closing time. Off to public transport again, arrive home, relax for a bit and then grab some dinner. Maybe some pasta tonight or pizza or just a cup of tea and off to bed, that's it. That's my day. Still why did the weight start to pack on? I mean I wasn't eating badly? Was I? Turns out I was.

A few searches on the internet and I realized I needed to do something new. What could that be though? Strangely enough I came across a book I had bought years ago. You know these old books you get at a garage sale or flea market. Apparently it turns out that I had one of those books and I have no clue at which point, in my especially busy life that I purchased it. It was an old book and I did edit the info a bit, you know, to suit my busy schedule. It worked for me but don't think it is a weight loss cure. It only gets the body started.

It turns out that in order to lose weight or more precisely body fat, at first a detox is important since toxins the body builds up are somehow associated with fat storage. Don't quote me on this but from what I understand if the body is too saturated with toxins, you know, from what we eat and drink on a regular basis, not to mention bad sleeping habits, stress and certain late night social activities, which have us out till we hours of the night, the body deals with this by storing body fat to trap the toxins and prevent them from damaging our internal organs. Wow, the body is smarter than I thought. So the theory is, if you detox the body, the fat now has no reason for being there and will begin to break down. If we include certain activities to increase our metabolism and encourage elimination of those toxins, namely exercise, it will make it easy to burn the fat in future as we progress to a more healthy and structured way of eating. Trying to lose weight without a detox may release these toxins into the blood and could put your organs at risk, so I decided to detox first.

Certain foods and food combinations are good for detoxes and certain ones aren't. Sometimes a good one can turn to a bad one if we ignore how we use them. The detox I used was a seven day fruit and vegetable detox. Since it is a detox we should avoid certain foods that can cause a buildup of toxins. Food products such as meat, yes, including fish, dairy and starches should be avoided for seven days.

On the last day of the fruit and vegetable detox I did a juice fast. Once again it is said that doing a liquid fast can help fat loss and help the body eliminate toxins as well as increase the production of certain hormones which are good for health but as we know these can be called theories. I will let you be the judge. On the next page I will have the fruit and vegetable detox and specific instructions I used. During this time I performed 1 hour of cardio a day be it running, walking, swimming, cycling or treadmill.

Try to keep active and avoid working too hard because it may be too much for the body since we are not eating from all food groups. More isn't always better.

7 Day Fruit and Vegetable Detox

Things to eat

- Unrefined food such as whole grain cereals, bran, honey, molasses, and lentils; green leafy vegetables, especially spinach, French beans, tomatoes, lettuce, onion, cabbage, cauliflower, Brussels sprouts, celery, turnip, pumpkin, peas, beets, asparagus, carrot; fresh fruits, especially pears, grapes, figs, papayas, mangoes, grapefruit(with fleshy area), gooseberries, guava and oranges ; dry fruits such as figs, prunes, raisins, apricots and dates ; fats in the form of nuts, peanuts, almonds, cashews, walnuts; oils such as virgin coconut oil, virgin olive oil, avocado and avocado oil.

Things to avoid

- Sugar and sugary foods should be strictly avoided because sugar steals B vitamins from the body, without which the intestines cannot function normally. Foods which constipate are all products made of white flour, white rice, white bread, pulses, cakes, pastries, biscuits, cheese, fleshy foods, preserves, white sugar and hard-boiled eggs. Most fruits are beneficial however avoid banana and jack fruit. The fast is a no meat fast so protein is restricted to nuts like almonds, peanuts, walnuts, etc.

Advice

- The above set of foods (things to eat) should be taken for 7 days and on the seventh day a twelve hour juice fast is preferable since this will maximize fat burning as well as clean the colon(orange juice is especially good for fasts). This means that if you wake up at 8:00am your fast ends at 8:00pm.
- Food should be properly chewed; each morsel for at least 15 times. Hurried meals and meals at odd times should be avoided.
- Water should be drunk half an hour before or after meals as it may dilute the stomach acid.
- Before bed try to eat either a bran based food (raisin bran is good) or a fruit.

- Bael fruit, pear, grapes, prunes and raisin are good for clearing the colon, soak prunes or raisins in water to give them their natural size, eat the fruit and drink the liquid before bed or after breakfast.
- Adequate exercise is especially preferable during this diet although one should try not to make it too strenuous, as such stick to cardio as recommended by this program.
- Plenty of water should be drunk at least 6 to 8, 8 ounce glasses a day (increasing of course during exercise). Make sure to eat till you are full at each meal as fruit tend to metabolize quickly leaving you hungry more often. Avoid starvation as this is not a starvation or crash diet, it is a detox and colon cleanse.

Sure, this detox may be difficult to follow and some of us need a more structured method since, yes, this can be a bit troublesome to look at. I mean, try looking at it pinned on your fridge while rushing out, so not happening. This is why I came up with a sort of meal plan for it. Okay, I know I am not a professional but I needed the structure, it just made sense to me. Below has the structure that you need and I put in the list of foods for good measure, you know, to make it easier on the fridge viewers.

Fruit & Vegetable Detox Meal Plan

Breakfast Between 7:00am - 9:00am	Snack Between 10:00am - 11:00am	Lunch Between 12:00pm - 2:00pm	Snack Between 3:00 pm - 5:00pm	Dinner Between 6:00pm - 8:00pm
3 to 5 servings of fruit/veg Include hot cup of green tea or herbal tea	1 to 2 servings of Nuts e.g. Peanuts or Almonds	3 to 5 servings fruit/veg ,1 cup of green tea	1 to 2 servings of Nuts e.g. Peanuts or Almonds	2 to 3 servings of fruit/veg, 1 cup herbal tea

- 1 serving of fruit and/or veg is equal to 1/2 cup, a portion equal to half the palm of your hand or 10 grams as read on nutrition labels. Make sure to understand the servings and usage of it in order to consume the right quantity of food.

- In the event of hunger it is fine to increase your meal by a serving especially if hunger persists. To avoid binging or to deal with sudden cravings always carry some prunes, raisins or nuts with you to keep you on track.

- 1 hour of cardio a day is recommended for this meal plan. 4 to 5 times a week is ideal. Avoid doing weight training, high intensity training or resistance training during this plan.

Foods to Eat

Whole Grain	Fat	Fruit	Vegetables
Amaranth	Brazil Nuts	Apple	Asparagus
Whole grain oats	Hemp seeds & oil	Berries	Bell/sweet peppers
Whole grain rye	Pine nuts	Cantaloupe	Cucumber
Buckwheat	Sesame seed & oil	Currants	Kale
Whole grain barley	Cashew	Dates	Lettuce
Brown rice	Walnuts	Grapes	Mushrooms
Quinoa	Avocado & oil	Limes/lemons	Olives
	Coconut oil	Mango	Parsley
	Olive oil	Melons	Sea Vegetables
	Grapeseed oil	Orange	Squash
	Almonds	Papaya	Onions
	Peanuts	Peach	Tomato
		Pineapple	Egg plant
		kiwi	Celery
		Guava	Cabbage
		Prunes & Raisins	Turnip
		Sour sop	Zucchini
		Tamarind	String beans

- **Nut milks are fine to consume especially with grain cereals, at the respective times which should be limited to no later than 2:00 pm, except on the last day where you do juice fast and can end the fast with them.**

- **A small amount of raw grains can be eaten with your nuts. Limit or avoid using grains that need to be cooked during the 7 days. Grains can be used only if the hunger is really bad, otherwise try to stick to what is listed in the Fruit and Vegetable Detox meal plan.**

What should I expect from following this? Well, I can't speak for everyone but I can say what I felt. I felt an increase in energy within the first two days. No longer did I feel gloomy and low. Not to mention the hour of cardio a day really helped boost my mood and made it feel like it was worth it. I felt like I was doing something good. My skin began to clear up, now I understand why they call fruit and vegetables glow food because that is how my skin looked and felt by the fourth day.

I knew something was going on inside of me because I had to do the "number two" more often and not in an uncomfortable way. It was easy and relaxing, sorry about this but I have to give my experiences, I know we are talking about poop but you know, we all do it, right? The hardest part for me was having a bowl of fruit and vegetables for lunch and watching people around me with their regular food. It's crazy! Why do you decide to eat fried chicken on the day I am eating fruit? Is this punishment for trying to clean up or is this a test of will power? Well, I passed that test and so can you.

The seventh day was the juice fast. This was probably the toughest part of the entire week. I mean we are talking about drinking watered down juice with minimal or no sugar at all. How did I get past it? Every time I felt hungry I filled my tummy with my diluted juice mixture. It helped a lot but be prepared to run off to do number one very often. If it comes out light yellow or clear you are on the right track. Yes, again, we are talking about pee. Hey, we've got to be open and honest about our functions, that is life people.

At the end of my fast, in the evening I ended it with a light soup broth, chicken or fish broth is fine maybe a little bit of the protein in there just for good measure, hey we earned it, right? Before I started the next level I had lost about 5 pounds, individual results will vary but expect to lose two to five pounds if you followed it perfectly. Be honest with yourself, it is your health, hold yourself accountable and take responsibility, the only one who can benefit from it is you and you alone, you deserve the best and this is you taking it.

Oh and for the ladies, if that dreaded time of the month is near and you feel heavy and bloated don't fret, it will pass, give it time, you aren't gaining weight. There is a theory that during that dreaded time ladies put on five to ten pounds of water. Don't worry about it, keep going, have some ginger tea, it helps some people but no matter what you do avoid the scale till after it is completely gone. It will kill your motivation. Remember, you are beautiful and wonderful every day of every month, girls are awesome!

Are you ready for the next level? I know I am. God, I am about done with this fruit thing, I mean come on, give me some meat, some potatoes, right? That's what I thought though, I am human. What about you? Write down what you felt in the notes section on the next page. See you at level 2.......

Record Your Goals 2

Current weight: _______________________________________

My experiences: _______________________________________

____

____

Words of Encouragement: ________________________________

____

____

____

____

Level 2

Fat Loss

Hi there, Tammey again. Hope you've been doing well. What a ride, right? I thought it would never be over but it has only just begun. Level 2 is about fat loss. Already? Well yes, we worked hard, so might as well start now. You have detoxed so now the body is ready to drop the fat it no longer needs. We finally get to eat real food again, right? Felt like a rabbit for a bit, not to knock people who enjoy that type of life style but let's face it, it is hard. Anyway, time to move on.

I won't lie and call myself a social butterfly but sometimes I like to go out a bit with a few friends. I mean, I don't have many friends but a small group of close knit people from days' past, like from college or something, the ones you gelled well with. You know, we perhaps go to a movie or even out dancing, maybe have a few drinks. However, I noticed something very strange. Whereas in the past a few drinks would have done me nothing to shout about, now I can hardly handle half a beer. Like, what's that about? Turns out that alcohol of any kind puts some of the toxins we just got out, right back. I mean, after only 1 week, really? I learned my lesson. Next time some fruit juice will have to do. My friends will just watch me oddly for a bit until they realize I am serious. Thankfully they were encouraging and made sure I did not drink.

You see, my friends, family and general social environment played a big part in my journey to better health. I like my friends, they held me accountable and it really helped me stay on track. In fact they all wanted to try the process when I was done, it was really cool. I'm telling you, make sure you have people around you that are supportive of your goals, it makes a huge difference. I never would have done it if it weren't for my support. Lesson learned. I won't be drinking anything but water and fruit juice again though. Not really interested in self-sabotage.

Back to the game plan! After level 1 your body is now in an environment where it will be happy to lose fat, if we give it the right encouragement. I remember, quite some time ago, reading a book about some guy who went to the mountains in Asia somewhere and met some monks. There he found that the monks all looked really young. Most of them looked like they were in their late twenties to early thirties with the occasional forty year looking guy. Imagine this; no one was under fifty years old. Seriously!

They welcomed him, of course, and they took him in for a bit. He worked with them, observing their habits, like tending to the fields but most importantly he noticed their eating. These monks did not eat like we do. You know our meats; our starches and a little dash of garnish that we like to call salad. No, these guys ate one food group at a time. They ate meat all by itself, most times one meat, at another time they ate their starches only and at night they mostly ate really light, like some vegetables.

Their reasoning for this was that eating different foods all at once kind of confuses the body and makes it harder on the stomach. I did some digging again, turns out, they were kind of right. Meat, starches and fats all digest at different rates and some even compete with each other. So for average Joe's and Jane's like us it makes it harder to lose weight. Did I mention they were all fit looking and strong? Well sure, they were monks and they did not have to worry about the stress of inner city living but it still held merit to me.

 Their eating was very efficient for their activity levels and so since their body did not need much to survive they just kept off the unneeded fat. Of course, that method won't work for me, not for someone who loves their food. Are you nuts? However, I did want to try something out, so I got to working and experimenting and what I came up with seemed to work for me.

What I did was divide my food up into portions and I made sure to always include vegetables with each meal. At breakfast I ate my protein with plenty of vegetables, according to some fitness specialists eating high protein foods in the morning, coming out of the long fasting period of sleep, helps you burn fat since the body is looking for protein. It usually gnaws away at the fat since the body tries to hold on to muscle, which is of course, made of protein and at our activity level it would be just enough, kind of like the monks.

The vegetables are important as well, as much as I hate them, they give you the vitamins and minerals to function, not to mention good dietary fiber. My research shows that meat based foods and processed starches have little or no fiber at all and can stay in the gut for quite some time. This would cause the body to get clogged and toxins may build up. The vegetables prevent this by helping the gut to push stuff down and out, you know, number 2. So a happy gut means fat loss.

 At lunch time would be a healthy starch source like whole grain bread, brown rice or maybe sweet potato. There are a whole host of healthy starches to choose from. Avoid sugary, processed starches like white flour and as much as I loved Irish potatoes I had to cut it back. Don't get me wrong, they are great but won't help much in this case. Starch is needed since the brain works on sugar but we need to get the healthy stuff that would encourage fat loss.

Since we did not eat starch at breakfast it is possible that by lunch we would feel tired and might lose focus. I know I got a real kick when I had lunch and for sure I did not have the sleepy feeling I usually have. I felt more energetic and kind of happy, it's strange but it worked for me so I tried to keep it up.

What really got me though, are the cravings for sugar and you know at that time coworkers are coming to work with donuts and chocolates. I mean, like seriously?

I'm working here people! Try to hold out on eating junk food around me, sheesh. I found that some fruit between breakfast and lunch and maybe a little, a few hours after lunch really helped cut the cravings but I stuck to prunes and raisins. They were more affordable for me, they helped the cravings and they were good for my gut, so I killed three birds with one arrow. Or is it stone? Whatever, it helped, that's what counts.

Dinner was probably the most disappointing. Remember, I used to have pasta or maybe pizza for dinner. Well that changed, can't say I was ecstatic about it but hey, if I'm going to do this, I might as well do it right and stick to it. I just had a light soup with maybe some chicken or fish floating around in it. No starch, a few vegetables though. Never have I ever loved vegetables so much. It's like the vegetables became the new potato and as you may notice, I love potatoes but sadly I had to avoid them.

On occasion I might have had some cereal but only a small bowl and I made sure to remain healthy, raisin brand or raisin oat bran were my cereals of choice but remember to stick to whole grain cereals, avoid the sugary stuff, no seriously, avoid it! Do you know how much I wanted a bowl of Lucky Charms? Also, get a nut-milk like almond milk or something, coconut milk is my all-time favorite. On the side I had maybe an egg or two, depending on my mood though. This is how I survived. Make sure you find what works for you while sticking to the plan.

This went on for the better part of three weeks. So, the question is "What exercise did you do during that time?" I simply doubled my cardio. The reason for this is the encouragement I mentioned earlier. For my body to lose the fat after doing the detox, I needed to encourage it to. I was now eating some protein so my muscles would recover and I would lose fat but I wasn't eating enough protein to train like, super hard, so this was how I pushed my body.

To be honest I really could not do more than that and let me tell you it worked like a charm. I saw significant changes in my body and yes I lost weight. Expect to lose body fat and to see your body changing but only if you do it perfectly, I mean like a monk, right, see what I did there? Tammey got jokes! Ok, that was corny, humor me.

There is one down side to this though. It's in the way I lost the fat. I noticed my legs, arms and neck were getting smaller, even my face a bit but the tummy was still there, I mean it was going down but not fast enough. For that brief time I remembered that I had been doing things badly for years I can't expect a miracle in a few weeks, it would take time. It seems, however that this is the way it is supposed to happen. Losing fat healthily starts from outward to inward so I was right on track and that gave me the will to keep going. On the next page I will give you the meal plan I used for this level as well as the list of foods.

Fat Loss Meal Plan

Breakfast Between 7:00am-9:00am	Snack Between 10:00 am-11:00am	Lunch Between 12:00 pm-2:00 pm	Snack Between 3:00pm-5:00pm	Dinner Between 6:00pm-8:00pm
1 to 2 servings of a Protein source e.g. Tofu, fish, chicken, egg, etc. With Raw fruit, and or vegetables and fresh fruit juice unsweetened or minimal sugar. Coffee or tea is permitted unsweetened or minimal sugar.	Fruit	1 to 2 servings of a Starch source like, brown rice, ground provision, etc with raw vegetables and or fruits and fresh juice minimal sugar. (one of the above, not all at once, with your greens)	Fruit	Light soup, or cereal with small amounts of protein and fresh fruit juice.

- Make sure to drink plenty of water and to eat plenty of fresh fruit and vegetables. Pace yourself, try to avoid over indulgence.

- 1 serving of protein or starch is equal to one cup, a portion equal to the palm of your hand or 20 grams as read on nutrition labels. Make sure to understand the servings and usage of them in order to consume the right quantity of food.

- Avoid mixing your starches at meals, try to use one starch source at a time

- This meal plan is designed to cause your body to burn food more efficiently which will in turn cause fat loss, another meal plan may be needed afterward to burn the fat which remains since at that point your body's metabolic rate would respond better to food.

- 2 hours of cardio a day is recommended for this meal plan. 4 to 5 times a week is ideal. Avoid doing weight training, high intensity training or resistance training during this plan.

Foods to Eat

Protein	Starch	Fat	Fruit	Vegetables
Eggs	Oatmeal	Nuts	Variety	Variety
Chicken	Whole wheat or Whole Grain Bread	Olive Oil	oranges	Spinach
Turkey	Whole grain Pasta	Flax seed	grape fruit	carrots
Lean Beef	Quinoa	Flax Oil	apples	broccoli
Lean Pork/Lean Ham	Sweet Potato	Hemp seeds or oil	pears	cauliflower
Fish	Grain Cereals	Avocado	grapes	lettuce
	Brown Rice	Fish Oils	kiwi	tomatoes
	Legumes		berries	cabbage
	Ground provisions		pineapple	Chinese cabbage
	Green Banana		melons(all)	local vegetables
	Bread Fruit		local fruit	etc
			etc	

This "Foods to Eat" list is very important. At times we get tired of eating the same thing over and over and this just gives you an idea of what foods to stick to in order to remain on track. If it isn't in the list you should avoid it. One food that is misunderstood is banana. Don't get me wrong bananas are very good but this is a fat loss level. I have noticed that bananas can reduce your ability to lose fat due to their high carbohydrate content and lack of fiber. They are good for recovery but it can cause a bit of a bloat, of course this is my experience and may not be yours. Play it safe and avoid it just for now.

So Tammey , what should I expect to see from this level? Well my energy levels remained high and I was quite happy with my body's changes. As long as you know what results to look for you won't feel discouraged. Just remember to look at your arms and legs and not your mid-section, that is the last to go. Another thing to pay attention to, and you need to be careful because it takes you off guard, it's your appetite, it goes through the roof at times and sometimes, you just don't feel to eat at all. Still eat though and in times of cravings know what you want.

Pace yourself. We all make mistakes and may falter at times but just forgive yourself, pick yourself up and keep moving forward. Don't let one bad meal or bad day mess up all your hard work and don't think that one good day is enough to get the results you are looking for. We are doing this one for three weeks so try your best to get in at least 5 great days each week.

A little tip to consider with your cardio, remember we are doubling it to two hours of cardio, try to mix it up, don't just do two hours on a treadmill, or a stationary bike. What I did was a cool brisk walk for one hour, either outside or on the treadmill then I split it up between a stationary bike and an elliptical or ski machine, those are the ones my neighborhood gym had, so those are the ones I used.

To mix it up a bit I did them in intervals. You know fast for a bit then slow and picked up the pace as my stamina got better. If it's too tough for you get a gym buddy or a trainer to push you through. You can do it! Stick to it, hold yourself accountable, believe in yourself and see you at level three!

Record Your Goals 3

Current weight: ____

My experiences: ____

____

____

Words of Encouragement: ____

____

____

____

____

Level 3

Fat

Burning

It's me again, Tammey. So you must be wondering, "Why is this level called fat burning?" Wasn't level 2 called fat loss? I suppose it's a matter of perspective. It's kind of like the difference between taking a shirt off and ripping it off. Taking off a shirt, well a loose fitting t-shirt, requires very little effort. You lift it over your head and drop it to the floor. Ripping a tight fitted shirt off requires actual effort and stress. I mean you really got to use that elbow grease to tear the thing off. Do you know how hard it is to do an incredible hulk or Hulk Hogan styled t-shirt rip. That is really hard work!

Well that is the difference between fat loss and fat burning in my opinion. Fat loss, to me, is making a few changes and doing some minor work to lose some fat, it kind of just appears to drop off but fat burning actually requires some muscle work. While it won't be hard work right off the bat, it will still be different compared to the other levels. To fully explain and understand this level I had to ask my fitness friend for a little help.

Do you remember from the previous levels, me mentioning doing research? Well asking my friend was part of that research. In the interest of privacy let's call him "Volt". Volt is a personal trainer and specializes in fitness nutrition and will be offering his expertise in the explanation of the methods I used in this level. According to Volt, fat loss can be described as the body using up its fat stores due to a change in diet or increase in cardio activity, which really is what we did in the first two levels. Isn't it?

Fat burning, he says, would be the act of actively engaging in activity which builds muscle and forces the body to use up further fat stores in order to build that muscle. The increase of muscle will also increase the amount of fat the body is able to burn. This is why this level is called "Fat burning". We're ripping the shirt people!

We will build a little more muscle, no you will not look like a man ladies, and that muscle will help us burn fat and improve our overall shape and appearance. Of course our focus is going to be the eating, since it is the hardest part but I will give you some guidelines for approaching the workouts with some help from Volt.

What I really loved about this part of my journey was it allowed a bit more freedom. I mean, I get a cheat day. A day I can eat whatever I want? Hello, hell, to the yes please! At last something I can follow. This is the day you can eat whatever you love or feel like eating. Of course, we still have to be careful and try not to overdo it but after all that hard work it was well worth the wait. Plus, why would I even bother sabotaging my hard work, I just want one day I can eat regular potatoes and cheese cake, sorry I love cheese cake. I can ignore everything else but cheese cake was the hardest thing for me to let go of. It might not be cheese cake for you but whatever it is, you finally get the chance to indulge. Sadly, you still need to avoid alcohol.

This meal plan uses the same list of foods but it is organized differently. Who knew that the order of food made a difference when trying to lose weight? Volt says this meal plan takes into consideration several methods in order to get the body to burn fat. Using his assistance I will explain to you the methods he mentioned.

The meal plan encourages you to increase your protein, doing so can increase your metabolism and allows your muscle to recover properly since the faster and better your muscle recovers, the more effectively you can burn fat. You will eat from a clean but good protein source 3 times for the day, breakfast, lunch and dinner. You will also have two snacks that should consist of nuts like almonds or peanuts and dried fruit like prunes or raisins, just like the previous level. This means I was eating 5 times a day. Volt says that this takes advantage of what is called the "thermic effect of food". Basically a fancy way to a say that your temperature goes up when you eat and so you can burn more fat, since you are hotter, literally.

There is also a cut off time for eating regular fruits, dried are still ok at a certain time. Apparently after two o'clock in the afternoon the body deals with sugar differently. Something about how our bodies react to the sun and we burn less fat as the sun goes down. The only exception would be the prunes and raisins since they help clean up the large intestine in the gut and a clean gut means better fat loss.

A few sour fruits can be eaten in the evening like green apples or grape fruit but still should be avoided. Instead, at night, I ate a protein source like chicken or fish with some vegetables. I liked fresh tossed salad, no pun intended, since I'm lazy and it was easier to prepare. I just chopped up some lettuce, cabbage and tomatoes and I'm good to go, sometimes just the lettuce or cabbage, again laziness. From what I understand, what this does is allow the body to chew on its own body fat while we are asleep and we won't lose much muscle since the training makes your body want to keep the muscle and repair it. The thing with muscle is that if it is being used you won't lose it.

Lastly the type of starch we eat is different. We should eat stuff like sweet potato, brown rice or quinoa, a strange one, I know, it's similar to rice and high in protein. The starches contain fiber and are what Volt calls slow burning starches, so your body burns it over a longer period of time and this keeps your temperature up and the fat keeps burning.

There is so much to this fat burning thing, like you have to go to school to understand it. Wait, you do have to go to school to understand it. Well for those who did not study fitness, get a trainer or fitness professional to explain it. Now, on to the training!

The training was simple as well and works better if you can join a gym or get a trainer that knows what to give you to do. Cardio would be just one hour, distributed however you choose but remember to do enough to adequately warm up and enough to cool down. The work out would not need to be very long, between thirty and forty five minutes is fine. Volt recommended that I worked a different muscle from each muscle group each day, to allow the entire body to burn fat while not over training.

Over training leads to injury, especially being a newbie. We can make it more challenging as we improve. He recommended doing 12 to 15 repetitions for 3 sets for all the areas trained for the day and by the end of the week the entire body would have been trained. He stresses using perfect form and breathing properly as well as drinking plenty of water. It is recommended that you get a trainer but if you are confident that you can do it yourself feel free to do so. Be creative and have fun.

The meal plan is on the next page and the list of foods remains the same. There is also a list of fitness supplements that I took that Volt recommended they are essential to preventing injury and increasing recovery.

Specific Fat Burning Meal Plan

Breakfast Between 7:00am-9:00 am	Snack Between 10:00am-11:00 am	Lunch Between 12:00pm-2:00 pm	Snack Between 3:00pm-5:00pm	Dinner Between 6:00pm-8:00pm
1 to 2 servings of Protein, 1 to 2 servings of whole grain bread or oats, with a fruit. Include hot cocoa, a green tea or decaffeinated coffee	1 serving of Nuts e.g. Peanuts or Almonds & dried fruit example prunes or raisins	1 to 2 servings of Protein, 1 serving of brown rice, or whole grain pasta, or sweet potato, with plenty of vegetables, 1 cup of green tea	1 serving of Nuts e.g. Peanuts or Almonds & dried fruit example prunes or raisins	2 servings of Protein, with plenty of vegetables, 1 cup herbal tea

- **1 serving of protein or starch is equal to one cup, a portion equal to the palm of your hand or 20 grams as read on nutrition labels. Make sure to understand the servings and usage of them in order to consume the right quantity of food. Fruit and veg would be 1/2 cup.**

- **In the case of vegetarians protein should be taken up to 3 servings as many sea based protein sources aren't as dense as land based ones.**

- **A serving of eggs is suggested at 3 eggs however females may start at 2 eggs and work their way up to 3.**

Foods to Eat

Protein	Starch	Fat	Fruit	Vegetables
Eggs	Oatmeal	Nuts	Variety	Variety
Chicken	Whole Grain Bread	Olive Oil	oranges	Spinach
Turkey	Whole grain Pasta	Flax seed	grape fruit	carrots
Lean Beef	Quinoa	Flax Oil	apples	broccoli
Lean Pork/Lean Ham	Sweet Potato	Hemp seeds or oil	pears	cauliflower
Fish	Grain Cereals	Avocado	grapes	lettuce
	Brown Rice	Fish Oils	kiwi	tomatoes
	Legumes	Coconut oil	berries	cabbage
	Ground provisions		pineapple	Chinese cabbage
	Green Banana		melons(all)	local vegetables
	Bread Fruit		local fruit	etc
			etc	

- While a healthy meal plan is good, it has its limitations and therefore variety is needed. In the event of the desire for meal variety this lists the best foods.

- Oil such as olive oil or flax seed oil should not be cooked at high temperatures. If cooking is required it is best recommended that you use coconut oil.

- Fish oil or omega fatty acid supplements are available at your local drug store or supermarket.

<u>Supplements Needed</u>

At this level training becomes very intense and the body uses up a great deal of Vitamins and Minerals. To prevent deficiency and injury the following supplements are the basics required to meet your nutrition requirements.

Here is a list of supplements you will need to help you reach a healthier body profile.

<u>Multi-Vitamin</u>: Nowadays it is almost impossible to get the nutrients we need from food alone especially for the training you will be engaged in so this supplement is needed. Take once daily.

<u>B-Complex</u>: Your body needs these for metabolic processes, especially B-12. This will aid with blood metabolism and overall cell regeneration.

<u>Fish Oil/Omega 3/Omega3/6/9</u>: This supplement can be taken in capsule form and will aid metabolism, reduce inflammation, increase circulation, aid mental alertness and improve general health and is a staple when it comes to supplements.

<u>Calcium/Calcium Citrate with D</u>: Especially needed to help alleviate osteoporosis. It is also needed for joint and cartilage repair, helps maintain these areas and protect them from shock and the wear and tear of training.

<u>Whey Protein</u>: A whey protein Concentrate or Isolate can be used to improve recovery and fat loss at this time. While not absolutely necessary it may greatly improve overall performance. For best results take no more than 45 minutes after your day's work out, the sooner, the better.

This meal plan I did for about four to five weeks and I did full body routines with light to moderate resistance. A resistance light enough to do with ease but heavy enough to offer a comfortable challenge. As I got stronger I increased the weight and sometimes the repetitions. It is very important to get your cardio in every day. I did thirty minutes before and thirty after to make up my hour but you can do it however you choose, just get it done.

Me, being the lazy person that I am, I will admit, I did not do super hard work for the strength training but I used a multi-station cable machine at my local gym. You know the machine with all the cables and pulleys and plates and stuff, not sure of the technical terms.

I will warn you that if you are expecting some miracles at this level you would be mistaken. I didn't lose much weight maybe three to five pounds. Perhaps if I had pushed harder but I was being my lazy self. I did notice a huge shape change and my clothes especially at my waist became very, very loose. I even had pants falling off but very little change on the scale. Volt told me that this meal plan would increase your muscle mass at the same time you lose body fat, so if I lose five pounds of fat I would gain five pounds of muscle and muscle taking up less space than fat, I would become trimmer.

Once again I got an increase in energy and I became stronger. I also noticed that I powered through my work out faster as time went by. If I had really put in the work I could have lost up to eight pounds though, and so I kept that in mind and decided that carrying forward I would hit it hard. I really became more motivated and the eating became easier. I was no longer craving the bad foods and I understood what my body needed when I got certain cravings, like craving for sweet foods meant I needed to up my protein. I also needed to up my protein if I had muscle soreness for more than two or three days, or I needed more sleep, getting seven to eight hours of sleep is ideal.

The most important part of this level is getting the meal plan and quantities almost perfectly during my training days and not over doing it on my cheat day. To be honest sometimes I didn't cheat, well I didn't feel I needed to, I don't know, perhaps I was really getting into this fitness thing. Now I would get people asking me if I was working out or if I am losing weight. I really started to realize how much people looked at me now that I am losing weight. I mean, people really like to mind other people's business but I guess that you are in public, so you are public eye property. Whatever happened to the rule that staring was bad? I guess that's just another unsaid rule out the window.

I will say that I did not experience joint pain and I was always mentally sharp and alert, this has to do with the list of supplements I was taking. They really helped at work as well and I was even happier to work there, well I appeared happier.

Who is happy to work, right? The snacks in between meals really helped a lot especially during the times I had the munchies or someone nearby had a food which was not on my list. It helped me stay current and I felt motivated and good about myself knowing that I was succeeding.

You see guys, not every time is the weight change a motivator, sometimes just knowing that you are doing the right thing for your health is motivator enough but we want results so health was not priority to me at the time. Volt said that weight is the least important measurement to follow in order to confirm fat loss and that investing in a measuring tape would be better. Taking measurements before and after gives a better idea of fat loss than the scale.

I will say you should avoid too many bananas, I mean seriously, I am not a fan of them but they really caused a bloat, I noticed the same with ripe plantain. It's not that they are bad to eat but they lack fiber and the time it remains in the gut is a bit delayed and can slow down movement for number two. I am not saying this is the case for everyone but it was the case for me. Tread the banana road with caution people.

Well we have made it this far and I know it was not easy but now we really get into the heat of the moment. The next level is when we can take it seriously. You can get a bit overwhelmed with this one but it is well worth it, trust me. See you later. I look forward to seeing you in the next level. Hopefully the last one right? You will have to read on to find out.

Record Your Goals 4

Current weight: _______________________________________

My experiences: ____

____

____

Words of Encouragement: _______________________________

____

____

____

____

Level 4

The Finale

Wow, you're back, you've made it this far so now we will be at, what for me, was the hardest part of my journey. This time I could not resort to my usual lazy self. I had to buckle down and buckle up because the ride became really a ride. It was downhill from here, really, I shit you not! If you think the other levels were tough, and for me they all were tough, then this one takes the cake. I really did feel for cake though. Anyway, back on track here Tammey, no more slacking off.

This level is where you can really tell if you want it or not. The eating wasn't something I was not already used to but I really had to put in the work with the exercise. I had to do a variety of exercises, I mean sure, I knew I could do it but sometimes I felt like giving up. My advice to you, get a training buddy, a trainer or even a coach. You can just get a good friend to edge you along, preferably someone who is focused on health, to prevent side tracking. This level is the last lap of the race. You know how runners really speed up for the last twenty meters? Well that is exactly how it's going to be here.

We have built enough muscle in the last level and now your body is a furnace. You eat your meals and snacks and you follow all the foods on your list down to the letter. Now we are going to let the furnace burn off the excess by adjusting our food a bit and increasing the intensity of the work outs. You may be wondering why we didn't just do this in the first place. Well firstly, a whole heap of things can go wrong if you just go from inactive to super active, it can range from joint issues, muscle damage, nausea, to even injury. Not to mention it's harder to stick to it and you can get discouraged if you are not really into exercise or have never done it before.

It can be very difficult to go right into the hard stuff and end up not doing so well. Makes you feel really bad about yourself and our body just isn't ready for it. Doing this gradually allows the body to make the needed changes and adjustments, it allows us to make mistakes and build good habits and taking this route allows us to stick with it long term. Many, and I mean many people, myself included, want to lose weight, get fit and be active but are worried that they won't be able to keep up. This is the main reason for this long method. Trust me it works and it feels good to, it really does.

So let's put our hard hat on and get right to it. For this level we still have to do one hour of cardio and we still do strength training but we kick in some high intensity interval training or "HIIT". What is high intensity interval training? HIIT for me is doing an exercise in short bursts of performance and then rest, usually for a certain amount of time, it can be any exercise. Here's an example, say I want to really burn out the thighs and butt, I could do squats as fast as I can for thirty seconds then rest for thirty seconds for say 6 sets.

There are many ways to do HIIT training but you should look into doing exercises that you like at first however you will need to aim for full body motions or at least work the entire body within a HIIT session. HIIT training is awesome since it puts your body in a fat burning state while allowing muscle building. In my research it creates what is called an "after burn" effect.

What this means is that your body continues to burn fat for up to two days after the workout. HIIT has one drawback though, it is hard on the joints so if you are going to do it every day break it up into different pieces, like you can do legs today, chest tomorrow, abs another day. If you are going to work all the muscles in one workout you should take the following day off from doing HIIT. Remember to take your supplements since it can be very draining and always remember perfect form.

The meal plan I used for this type of training is a very simple adjustment to the one from level 3, as I said, a minor adjustment. Simply remove starch from your lunch, yup, that's it. Similar to in level 2 it forces the body to use fat as energy since we reduced overall starch sooner. Breakfast remains the same with protein, starch and vegetables and dinner also stays as just protein and vegetables at night. Seems like an easy change right? Wrong, it is harder than you think!

You may feel hungrier and so you may have to max out your protein, perhaps increase your serving of nuts by about half a serving. For me, I really had to increase my protein for the main meals by about half a serving; I found that it worked better for me that way. Play around with it a bit, feel it out and see which one works best for you. I will leave the meal plan that I used on the next page. By now you would have figured out that the list of foods is the same, so I won't include it. Being the final stage, it will be easy to continue as things are.

Advanced Fat Burning Meal Plan

Breakfast Between 7:00 am - 9:00 am	Snack Between 10:00 am -11:00am	Lunch Between 12:00 pm - 2:00pm	Snack Between 3:00 pm - 5:00pm	Dinner Between 6:00pm - 8:00pm
1 to 2 servings of Protein, 1 to 2 servings of Starch, with 2 servings of Fruit. Include hot cocoa, green tea or herbal tea	1 serving of Nuts e.g. Peanuts or Almonds & dried fruit example prunes or raisins	1 to 2 servings of Protein, with 2 to 3 servings of vegetables, 1 cup green tea	1 serving of Nuts e.g. Peanuts or Almonds & dried fruit example prunes or raisins	1 serving of Protein, with 2 servings of vegetables, 1 cup herbal tea

- 1 serving of protein or starch is equal to one cup, a portion equal to the palm of your hand or 20 grams as read on nutrition labels. Make sure to understand the servings and usage of them in order to consume the right quantity of food.

- Please note that the hot cocoa mentioned above should be made without cow's milk. Straight hot water or an alternative like coconut milk is acceptable.

So what should we notice from this level you ask? There are a few things which are different that I noticed after four to five weeks at this level. I lost more weight, yes, of course, but that isn't the only thing. There was noticeable change in my shape, sure I did see a change of shape from level 3 but this was a whole other level. My clothes fit way looser and my tummy was noticeably flatter, I even saw the figure eight shape, you know the lines on either side of the tummy that runs down from the ribs down to the hip bone, yea that's the one.

My arms became more defined, not manly defined but toned, my legs were more firm. Over all I looked and felt better than I did before I started. Expect a further five to ten pound loss of body fat but that depends, of course, on how well you stick to the meal plan and how many days a week you trained. Don't expect miracles if you only punched out two or three days a week. If you put in the time and the grime you will be fine, trust me. There will always be more that can be done but if you came this far, be proud, you made it.

I spoke to Volt again and he said that after this level you can move from the meal plan in level 3 to this one and expect to quickly lose more. It is a very basic form of carb cycling where you add and remove starch in a way to trigger fat loss, it sure does work though, let me tell you. Volt also told me that it is possible to go even further, a possible level 5, if you will but it is way more advanced and would be great for persons interested in competitive fitness competitions and even sports athletes.

He said that you basically get a meal plan designed using your body type and this would super charge you to greater levels, you can get into the best shape of your life this way but it is completely personalized. For more information I will leave an email to contact Volt if you are interested.

Me, I'm not interested in going on stage or competitive sports, I just wanted to lose weight, get fit and feel better about myself and this worked for me. I hope it will work for you. I will continue to keep improving and watching my eating habits. I may indulge once in a while, on my cheat day but I won't over do it.

Other people took notice of my transformation, even my coworkers were surprised. Let this be our little secret. What do you say? Work hard, train smart and remember, no excuses! I can no longer say I'm old lazy Tammey, although the couch seems like a good place to be but it just doesn't feel right any more. Something about exercise makes you want to keep doing it. Know what I mean? Tammey Endevor, signing out, till next time, bye.

Oh yea, you can contact Volt at voltagefitness.vfslu@gmail.com. Say Hi for me, bye!

Record Your Goals 5

Current weight: _______________________________________

My experiences: _______________________________________

____

____

Words of Encouragement: _______________________________

____

____

____

Bibliography

Level 1:

Patrick, Rosalyn. Detox. New Lanark, Scotland. Geddes & Grosset, First Published 2002, reprinted 2003, 2005, printed and bound in Poland

Supporting research
Toxicological Function of Adipose Tissue: Focus on Persistent Organic Pollutants
Michele La Merrill, Claude Emond, Min Ji Kim, Jean-Philippe Antignac, Bruno Le Bizec, Karine Clément, Linda S. Birnbaum, Robert Barouki
Environ Health Perspect. 2013 Feb; 121(2): 162–169. Published online 2012 Dec 5. doi: 10.1289/ehp.1205485
https://www.ncbi.nlm.nih.gov/pmc/articles/PMC3569688/

Modulation of persistent organic pollutant toxicity through nutritional intervention: emerging opportunities in biomedicine and environmental remediation
Michael C. Petriello, Bradley J. Newsome, Thomas D. Dziubla, J. Zach Hilt, Dibakar Bhattacharyya, Bernhard Hennig
Sci Total Environ. Author manuscript; available in PMC 2015 Sep 1. Published in final edited form as: Sci Total Environ. 2014 Sep 1; 0: 11–16. Published online 2014 Feb 13. doi: 10.1016/j.scitotenv.2014.01.109
https://www.ncbi.nlm.nih.gov/pmc/articles/PMC4077968/

Level 2:

Kelder, Peter. Ancient Secret of The Fountain of Youth. Gig Harbor, Published by Harbor Press Inc, 1985, 1989 USA

Supporting research

Appleby, Maia. "What Are the Benefits of Lots of Protein in the Morning?" *Healthy Eating | SF Gate*, http://healthyeating.sfgate.com/benefits-lots-protein-morning-3574.html. Accessed 03 April 2018.

Heather J Leidy, Laura C Ortinau, Steve M Douglas, Heather A Hoertel; Beneficial effects of a higher-protein breakfast on the appetitive, hormonal, and neural signals controlling energy intake regulation in overweight/obese, "breakfast-skipping," late-adolescent girls, *The American Journal of Clinical Nutrition*, Volume 97, Issue 4, 1 April 2013, Pages 677–688, https://doi.org/10.3945/ajcn.112.053116

Important Basics Food Charts, Dietary Fiber http://apjcn.nhri.org.tw/server/info/books-phds/books/foodfacts/html/data/data2c.html

Effects of Food Processing on Dietary Carbohydrates: http://www.fao.org/docrep/W8079E/w8079e0j.htm

Tallmadge, Katherine. Eat More Early, Eat Less at Night https://www.livescience.com/45990-morning-meals-cut-evening-food-binges.html

Decker, Fred. "Do Some Foods Take Longer to Digest Than Others?" *Healthy Eating | SF Gate*, http://healthyeating.sfgate.com/foods-longer-digest-others-11622.html. Accessed 03 April 2018.

Level 3:
Supporting research

Specific Dynamic action/Thermic effect of food https://en.wikipedia.org/wiki/Specific_dynamic_action

Nauert PhD, R. (2015). 'Use it or Lose It' Is True for Muscle Mass. *Psych Central*. Retrieved on April 3, 2018, from https://psychcentral.com/news/2015/06/29/use-it-or-lose-it-is-true-for-muscle-mass/86225.html

John M. de Castro; The Time of Day of Food Intake Influences Overall Intake in Humans, *The Journal of Nutrition*, Volume 134, Issue 1, 1 January 2004, Pages 104–111, https://doi.org/10.1093/jn/134.1.104

Level 4:

<u>Supporting research</u>

Tao, David. How to Keep Burning Calories When Your Workout Is Over
<u>https://greatist.com/fitness/afterburn-effect-keep-burning-calories-after-workout</u>, *Originally published March 2012. Updated January 2016*

Stiehl, Christina. The Science Behind the Afterburn Effect
<u>https://www.shape.com/fitness/tips/science-behind-afterburn-effect</u>,
Mar 15, 2017

Mawer, Rudy. MSc, CISSN, What is Carb Cycling and How Does it Work?
<u>https://www.healthline.com/nutrition/carb-cycling-101</u>, June 12, 2017

Appendix

The Weight Loss Treatment Program

Level 1	Level 2	Level 3	Level 4
Detox	**Fat loss**	**Fat Burning**	**The Finale**
1 week	3 weeks	4 weeks	4 weeks
One week fruit and vegetable detoxification diet. Used to flush the body of toxins, begin the clearing process of the colon and alkalize the body.	Begins the fat loss process by making the body more efficient allowing the body to drop unwanted fat stores fast.	Puts your body in a fat burning environment allowing the building of just enough muscle to burn fat, tone up and trim down.	Uses the muscle from the previous level to amp. up your fat loss. Causes the body to really show the results of your training. More fat will be burned and your body will now become a fat burning furnace.
1 hr cardio daily	2 hrs cardio daily	1 hr cardio & strength training	1hr cardio, strength training & HIIT
7 Day fruit &Veg fast, meal plan	Fat loss meal plan	Specific Fat Burning Meal Plan	Advanced Fat Burning Meal plan

About the author

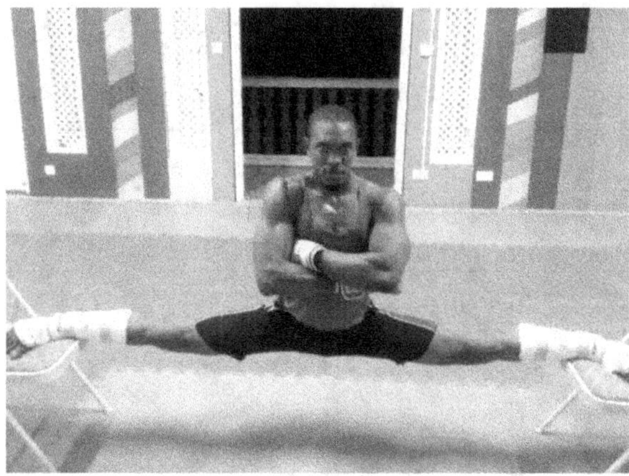

The Murray is a devout fitness enthusiast. Having started martial arts from the tender age of nine, he gravitated towards fitness and became drowned in it, finding a love that can compare only to his love for the fighting arts. He previously completed certification with ISSA (International Sport Sciences Association) as a Fitness Trainer and Specialist in fitness Nutrition and has since designed many workout programs and nutrition plans.

Having several black belts in martial arts and once having his own kick boxing club he wanted to share his love for fitness in his writing. Truly passionate about training and dedicated to his clients he seeks nothing short of the best for all with whom he comes into contact. With over 15 years of training experience he seeks, in his writing, to relate to the reader and to have the reader feel like they are part of the journey, following closely with his characters, which he creates from the several inspiring and influential persons he feels honored to have trained.

Feedback for this book may be directed to the.weightlosstreatmentprogram@gmail.com and persons interested in consultation, training or any general question about his work may be directed to voltagefitness.vfslu@gmail.com.

Acknowledgements

I would like to thank all my clients who over the years supported me and from whom I was inspired to write this work. Being the first of several to come, their continual support and their candid personalities allowed me the opportunity and the freedom to observe them and share with them, while assisting them with meeting their fitness goals, of which I feel honored. I also would like to thank the following individuals:

Miss Lavina D. Alexander
Bsc - Chemistry,
Msc - Water Resource Technology & Management

Miss Leona Sandra Phillip Murray
Bsc - Natural Sciences, Msc - Nutrition

Both of whom I am extremely grateful to for taking the time out of their busy schedules to go through my first work ,offering honest, clear and productive criticisms which not only helped me complete this work but also inspired me on this new journey that I have chosen to tread. I hope that in future they can grace me with their input and help enlighten my path as I continue forward.

I leave now a special thanks to two more persons. Of the two I would like to first thank Miss Laureen Fenelon. While several persons in the past may have suggested that I write a book, it was she who initiated the spark that led to this work. She edged me gently along with her advice, experiences and her cheerful demeanor. I am very happy that I was able to meet and work with her. It was truly a blessing.

The second of the two persons I would like to thank is Miss Deanna J. Dujon. My girlfriend and best friend, her encouragement and support gave me the confidence to allow me to think that I could do whatever I wanted to, no matter how hard. Constantly checking on the progress of this work and making sure I am consistent and focused. It is not often that we find, nowadays, a person who is as genuine and honest as she is, assisting not only with her presence but with her creativity and artistic input, thank you.

Lastly, I would like to close by thanking Miss Dawn French and Miss Kayra Williams, two fellow authors who are both encouraging and beautiful in personality and demeanor. While I only met them once at a publishing seminar,

Miss Dawn French being the presenter and Miss Kayra Williams being a fellow attendee, their drive to success kindled in me a desire to turn my whimsical dream into a reality.

At long last I thank the publisher but most importantly I thank you the reader. Without you none of this would be possible. I hope that my work reaches you, teaches you and inspires you to not only follow your dreams but to love and appreciate yourself and those around you. Always seek the best from yourself and give it to yourself. Continue to strive and grow in ways you never dreamed of. We can find inspiration all around us, let this inspiration fuel your life and make it forever fruitful and enjoyable.

Disclaimer

The information provided in this book is based solely on the opinions and experiences of the author. Taking into consideration the differences of individuals, purchasing this book confirms that you understand that results may vary and there is no guarantee that the claims made in this book will work for you. This book is not designed to provide helpful information on the subjects discussed and is not meant to be used, nor should it be used, to diagnose, treat or cure any disease or medical condition.

For diagnosis or treatment of any disease or medical condition, consult a trained physician. The publisher, author and any individual mentioned in this book are not responsible for any specific health conditions or allergies that may require medical supervision and are not liable for any damages or negative consequences from any treatment, action, application or preparation, to any person reading or following the information in this book.

References are provided for informational purposes only and do not constitute endorsement of any websites or other sources. Readers should be aware that the websites listed in this book may change and are not controlled by the author or any individual mentioned in this book.

www.ingramcontent.com/pod-product-compliance
Lightning Source LLC
Chambersburg PA
CBHW070056260726
48658CB00002B/889